Reader's Reaps

"What a wonderful read from start to finish! It felt like Jane was beside me telling me her story and encouraging me to join her to find the place of peace within. A daily message to comfort the soul with the wisdom of the ages supplying your daily bread of hope and peace that surpasses all understanding!"

--*Kathleen Caught,*
AMP, Accredited Mortgage Professional
President, Barrhaven Business Exchange
Author of *"From Marriages to Mortgages"*

"This book is an inspiration to anyone who wishes to expand their consciousness through meditation. Jane's gentle, non-judgemental approach to the subject matter allows one to consider the many different paths to meditation. She shares her personal experiences with an open heart that gently leads one to explore their own path."

--*Tashene Wolfe*
Teacher, Life Coach, and Author of *"A Path to Wholeness: A Spiritual Perspective on Understanding and Healing the Gaps in Your Life"*

"*In Silence* gives wise and gentle counsel to compliment and enhance our meditation process by gifting us with lovely insightful messages to focus upon during our daily meditation, and with helpful and clear suggestions to fine-tune our creative process of being still. I thought this little book would be a lovely gift to present to someone who is just starting to explore meditation, as well as for the seasoned meditator by supplying a new focus to their perceptions. By its mere simplicity it simply **IS.**"

--*Donna Doherty*
Stained Glass Artist, Reiki Master/Teacher, Aromatherapist

"There is extraordinary strength, wisdom and peace to be found in only a single moment of silence. Jane Rosalea Booth has created a simple but profound guide for exploring the gift of our inner sanctuary. *In Silence* is an inspirational carrying companion to personal meditation that invokes personal introspection and individual understandings. It reminds us to live each moment from the natural, peaceful place where we are closest to God. *In Silence* is a pure and beautiful book that comes from the heart. It holds wisdoms not to be missed."

--Rev. Dr. Marianne Zinn-Kuwabara
EMF Balancing Technique: Worldwide Support Team; Reiki Master

"This is an intimate account of the achieving of a personal journey, which finally leads to a new discovery of our nature and life. What makes this book so special is the simplicity of it. It doesn't force readers into any spiritual path. It doesn't offer any extreme changes in life. It just suggests some thoughts that may help our inner self to come outside and feel the world by itself without any prejudices, any rush or preconception. Going through the pages of Jane Rosalea Booth's book, the world suddenly appears as a calm place. I could feel an unusual strength inside of me making its way to my brain while I was reading it. Jane has created her technique by experiencing it on herself. She went through some personal difficulties in life and she felt she needed to explore her inner self to find braveness and confidence enough to help her in getting out of her own troubles. That's what makes this book such a good read and such a useful tool: the personal touch, the lack of complex methodology and just it being a real experience."

--Manuela Mesco
Publisher's review at www.in-silence.net

IN SILENCE

Discovering Self through Meditation

Jane Rosalea Booth

Cover Art by Eugenia Carroll Cusson

Illustrated by Elizabeth McNeil

To Ian, Andrew, Sarah and Bob

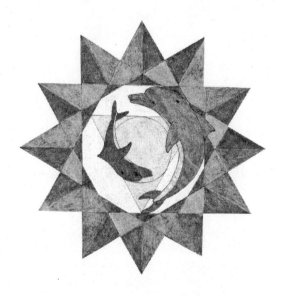

Contents

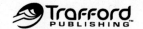

Acknowledgements

I give my heartfelt appreciation to those who have assisted and encouraged me in so many ways to create this book:

--To Eugenia Carroll Cusson, whose cover art so perfectly reflects the beauty of being in silence;

--To Elizabeth McNeil, for her generous hours creating beautiful graphics;

--To Lori South, for her editing and creative thoughts;

--To Michelle Jardin, for her support and editing;

--To James Twyman and fellow Ministers of Spiritual Peacemaking, for sharing the deep joy of peace and for being such a blessing in my life;

--To the participants of my Peaceful Path Holistic Meditation Workshops, for your awareness, inspiration, and laughter, I thank you;

--To Margaret Janecki, for her encouragement and loving friendship;

--To my husband Ian, my children Andrew and Sarah, Ian's family and my wonderful friends, who are always beside me.

In deepest gratitude, Jane

Part I

Discovering Self through Meditation

From the Silence Within

Discovering Self through Meditation

In 1987, I was sitting on a high hillside overlooking a lake near Kunming, China. I was alone, which was a rare occurrence during the three weeks I had been touring China with a group of YMCA volunteers. It was there, for a few breathtaking moments, that I captured a view of a most incredible sight. From my vantage point, I looked through some dark leafy trees to an opening where the sun was shining and reflecting upon the lake far below. I felt pulled from my dark, shadowy place into a beautiful, beaming light. Although I had seen this imagery in my meditations, I had never seen the symbolism of moving from the shadow into lightness so vividly in nature. This image came to me while I was experiencing some personal difficulties and this symbolism was the reminder I needed. There is always light beyond the dark shadows. Taking a deep breath, I soaked in the scene; closed my eyes and meditated . . . listening for guidance. The message I received from my meditation was "I must live my truth." This thought may seem simple, but it was the greatest, most awakening perception that I had ever had.

Imagine that a few moments of meditation on a hillside in China changed my life. It led me to making choices and decisions that changed my lifestyle and relationships. I moved from a wealthy, comfortable lifestyle into the life of a student, from a wife to a divorced woman who was alone, lonely and questing, from feeling unloved to eventually after several years, to experiencing a deep love. I was thirsting for more knowledge and the answer to the eternal question: "Who am I?" This thirsting was especially strong after my journey to China where I had just a taste of some of the ancient Chinese wisdom. When I returned, I enrolled at the University of Waterloo. As a forty-year-old among young people half my age, I felt uncomfortable and my fear of failing frightened me. It almost choked me from going on.

During the next two years of studies, I used meditation as a means to keep focused and to tap into my higher consciousness for guidance. I would meditate each morning and evening. After each meditation, I wrote what I called my "messages." I used short meditations before each exam along with some positive affirmations, and the results were shocking to me! I could remember most of what I had studied. Facts, formulae and ideas came to me easily as I wrote my examinations. Meditation helped me stay calm and clear under these stressful times.

Meditation now provides me with a shelter of protection, a place of peace and the courage to see each day as a *"beginning."* The messages in this book are a manifestation of my discoveries about love, daily life, nature and about the infinite beauty of our mysterious universe. It is in silence, the place of quiet stillness within, that I discover the truth of the loving essence of God, the Divine Spirit, who begins to merge with my inner self, and then becomes reflected in each moment of my life. I feel God as a complete whole -- both the Divine Masculine energy and the Divine Feminine energy -- in its purest unified form. It is from the experience of this wholeness that leads me from "seeking" for something to just "being" my true self. From this space, I am accepting and feeling blessed for all my experiences. I begin to look forward to new adventures and the unknown.

For over twenty-five years I have had some extraordinary spiritual experiences -- visions of angels, glowing orbs, sparkling bursts of lights -- showing me there are energies around me that are beautiful and comforting. As I meditate and listen to my inner consciousness, I hear my inner voice resounding messages that are full of words of encouragement, love and hope. I believe all of us have an inner consciousness that we can tap into to connect with universal energies and ultimately to our Divine Spirit.

During my meditation, I see spinning circles of colourful lights that whirl quickly to become a brilliant, white light. As I concentrate and merge with the white light, I often meet a guide called Rashna, a glowing white figure with a long beard wearing a white robe, who embraces me. I know many writers who connect with spirit guides are very definitive about whom their guides are. I heard the name Rashna in my meditations many years ago. I feel that Rashna is a guide of ancient wisdom and knowledge. He/she speaks using "ye" and "doth". Although I thought it was strange to hear this dialect, I have grown to enjoy the old English and have come to understand it as a sign that I must listen to these messages. Often, a group of white-robed people, similar to Rashna, surrounds me. I sense that these people are also sages or wise beings who are here to teach me. I also meet guides of wisdom called "Keepers" who provide ancient teachings about opening our gates of inner consciousness.

Other times, the vision is quite different with a group of people dressed in long Victorian gowns and fancy suits greeting me. This group loves to waltz! Sometimes I receive images of people dressed in 20th century clothing. Everyone is happy and peaceful! Each meditation presents new pictures and events to view, and most importantly, a place to listen for guidance. These visualizations are most loving, inspiring and awesome. What I am tapping into, I can assure you, is a source of love within me that is always with me, unfailing, unconditional, and eternal.

Often while meditating I feel a sense of weightlessness and floating with no sense of my body. It feels as though I am flying. Some may think I am dreaming, but I am not asleep nor in a trance during my meditations. I believe I move into a higher dimension, a higher consciousness that is just as much a part of me as my physical life is. However, the important point is that I become more aware of who I am and what I value and define as my truth when I move into the silence within me.

Why am I sharing these experiences now? The time has come for all of us to experience the loving union with our Divine Spirit. It is a time for us to become peaceful, to be peace. I believe that when we open ourselves and awaken our spiritual consciousness, our lives broaden and grow in ways that we can hardly imagine! Life is exciting and miraculous if we allow it to be. Each of us deserves to live without fears and to center ourselves in trust, love and joy. We have to remember what it is like to feel well, to feel happy and most of all -- to feel loved. I hope this book with its messages will help you recall those feelings.

Many write of transformation and the integration of our ego (our personality) with our soul. As we truly trust in Divine guidance, we feel the energies of love that surround us when we center ourselves in love. Then our lives transform, change and blossom. We end our separation from one another and from our spiritual source.

As you learn to meditate, a sense of connection to all of nature and the universe deepens and broadens, and you begin to see your life's purpose with greater clarity. You are very important. Each action and thought you create affects everyone else on this planet and in our universe. Your every choice, your every action is extremely significant to our movement towards a society whose actions are coming from the heart in love and forgiveness and not from the reactions of the ego based on fears, anger and hatred.

Yet, as I meditated, questions still haunted me and I continued to seek answers. How do I make the best choices and actions? What can I do to make my life wonderful and truly peaceful? What is my true life's purpose? In seeking these answers, I made several lifestyle changes in my relationships and my work. I went through many fear-based thoughts and anxieties that shook me to my core. Yet, each time when I had the strength to take a step forward, an unusual experience, new people or events entered my life to help redefine my beliefs, desires and values.

I discovered, as long as I stayed heart-centered, my life manifested in positive ways. However, if I did not, I found difficulty with financial challenges, relationships and at times, I felt overwhelmed with more fears. I would feel depressed, become ill and slip into my cozy "cave," as I called my bed. My illnesses gave me good excuses to be in my "cave" with my blanket pulled over me, and blinds closed to shut out the world. However, I was not enjoying these moments. I began, during these shadowy times, to meditate and to ask for help that I always received in many forms and ways.

The messages from my meditations encouraged me to give thanks and embrace both my shadowy (negative) times and my happy times. I really had to stretch with this concept, but now I look for the deeper meanings in difficult, unhappy events. This was not an easy task in times of trouble or illnesses of loved ones. Slowly, I moved into a place of forgiveness and more compassion for others from my past, as my perceptions of my life changed. I began to take responsibility for my previous actions and I stopped blaming others. My greatest leap in consciousness was in forgiving myself, ridding myself of guilt and frustration over seemingly failed relationships or work-related projects. Guilt stopped me from moving forward. It was truly stifling! I discovered that "everything has a purpose," a message my father gave to me as a young girl, but it took years to grasp this truth. Each happening moved me forward, increased my strength, and deepened my trust, love and alignment with God. This helped me to have new perceptions of my past, and to look forward with open eyes and heart.

Today, I try to live, to feel, to be fully present in this moment, the *now*. This can be a difficult task at times, but with a conscious effort, living in the *now* starts to become a way of life. I find it keeps me focused on my work and I am much more productive. The *now* is all we truly have and the more we embrace the present moment, the more we live fully and know our true being.

When I was a teenager, I thought that I was to meet a man, a soul mate, who would complete me. I had a yearning for a "perfect mate." Eventually, I realized that what I was seeking was to have a better relationship with myself and to learn how to love myself fully. I developed this relationship by allowing myself time to be in silence and to meditate daily. Most of us do not treat ourselves as our best friend or even think about treating ourselves well without feeling guilty. It took a long time for me to learn to treat myself as a good friend. I had to push past my old self-criticisms to find a person that I liked. As I became gentler and more forgiving with myself, this reflected more positively with my relationships with others. I stopped looking to others to define and approve of me.

What is so wonderful on my spiritual pathway is how life provides the very experiences that I need to move forward. However, I must keep my mind clear and my heart warm to receive messages. I see meanings in symbols in nature and my environment. I receive meaningful messages from everyone I encounter daily. Now, everything and everyone is important to me.

My meditations bring clarity to spiritual words and concepts. Here are my interpretations of some of the most significant images I have experienced.

God: Divine Spirit, Divine Creator, Divine Source, Love, Oneness

Angels: beauties of luminous light and love, breathtaking, awesome

Keepers: ancient ones who guide us, masters of great wisdom and knowledge

Scroll: a reminder of ancient teachings waiting to be recalled

Seasons: reflections of change, contemplation, movement and renewal

Garden: a safe place within, tranquility, peace, and harmony

Veil: the illusion that surrounds us, the masks we wear

Chalice: a holy vessel, a temple of peace, the womb

Combining visualization with meditation is a powerful tool that I use towards manifesting my desires. Each day, I visualize, with detail, all my desires. This creates a picture in my mind of a life full of abundance and joy. Even though the outer world seems chaotic, with meditation there is an inner sanctuary where I visualize my dreams. I receive a clearer focus and a sense of peace. Simple, easy-to-learn, and beneficial, meditation requires only a commitment of time for daily practice, a quiet place and a desire to experience a sense of spiritual connection -- a sense of Oneness with the Divine Spirit.

I believe the Divine Spirit only presents to us what we need and what we can handle. Each day brings new thoughts, new perceptions that make my life exciting and fulfilling ... a true adventure. During my meditations, I have the opportunity to move more deeply into my heart space. I stop controlling and humbly surrender to the Divine Spirit from a place of trust and deepest gratitude. I allow the Divine light to merge with me, healing and loving me, and showing me the way of peace. Everyone has an inner temple of wisdom with a voice of guidance and love. Do not hesitate to ask for help and guidance during your meditations. You will receive it. Use all your senses and intuition to expand your being and allow all your creative passions to emerge. Have no fears, as God, the Divine Creator, loves you. God sees your perfection, and only gives you messages of love. Here is one of the most powerful messages that I received in 1997 about love.

Love is the essence of life
The foundation
All that is
Ye cannot love one too much
If it is true compassion
Seek not love in return
Simply feel it from within
See it in each flower, each rainbow, each raindrop
Feel the loving energies of the universe surrounding you
Relax in the unknown
Harmony comes when conflict leaves
Seek the harmonious path
Ye are blessed; ye are protected
Ye will be led to wondrous places
Ye will do wondrous works
For the children, for the seekers
Live in thy truth of love
Ye are on the path leading to heightened awareness
Of universal love and joy

I would like to share with you the following messages from my meditations that I have recorded, with the words exactly as I heard them. Please join me as a fellow traveler who is becoming aware of your soul and your deep inner peace through greater spiritual connection and universal consciousness. I hope you will experience a new thought, feeling or sensation each time you open to a message. I invite you to reflect upon a message before you meditate. Ask your angel or guide for further clarity that relates to your life. We are all on this planet to learn the same truth, so my messages are for everyone. These messages are like kind words from a dear friend offering gentle advice, hope and love. Often I find new understanding of a message each time I read it, even years after I have written it.

After each meditation write your thoughts in a journal, record them on a tape recorder or draw a picture of your experience. These thoughts may not seem significant at this time, but soon their meanings will become clear to you. You will acquire a marvelous collection of your very own messages. They will be a source of guidance that you can enjoy during your lifetime. The messages that I receive today still leave me in awe and wonderment as they continue to open me to more cosmic awareness. They have evolved from messages about my personal human consciousness, to global consciousness, and now, to speak of cosmic consciousness.

It is so exciting to receive new ideas and concepts that I can contemplate and integrate into my life. I now understand there is nothing for me to seek as I already have all the tools -- the paint, the brushes and the canvas -- to create the life I want. These messages guide me gently into greater love and alignment with God's will.

There are many messages in this book for you to enjoy. In this section, *Messages of Love* will open your heart to love yourself and others fully. These messages guided me in times of darkness and led me to a place of peace. You may like to reflect upon a message before you meditate. In Part II, *A Daily Guide for Meditation and Self-reflection*, you will find easy steps to begin meditating and *Messages from the Garden Within* to contemplate daily. These messages contain spiritual concepts that can help you to be open to receive abundance, and to allow God's spirit to embrace you tenderly.   In Part III, *Nature's Guide to Spiritual Awareness* and *Messages of Wisdom* will increase your connection to all life. I especially love these messages as they hold the energy and ancient wisdom of each animal or plant they represent. In spite of the chaos we see on television and feel in our personal lives, we can still see the beauty of God's love in nature. Each one of us is special, with vast potential, many gifts and unique talents to share. Going into your silence in meditation will help you discover your life's purpose, create more love in your life as you expand your inner awareness, and allow the Divine Spirit to guide you. You will begin to find balance and wholeness in your daily life by releasing old patterns of fear and resistance that cause blockages to your success. You will only allow positive, loving thoughts into your consciousness. Your universe will expand and reflect back to you an abundance of love, prosperity and inner peace. From your awakened consciousness, your creative thoughts emerge! You can create the life you want!

Messages of Love

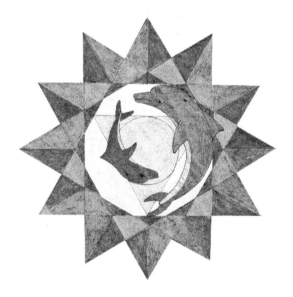

From the Sacred Heart

The Light shines beyond the shadow

Move gently, my child, with grace

Be peaceful, tranquil, and joyous

Dance in the merriment

Feel your heart song singing

Lifting you to new heights

Discard that which no longer serves

Be still, listen

In peace and serenity

In silence, for messages of love

"All is well"

All is as it should be

If it were not, so I would tell thee

Peace, child, fill with hope, love, renewal

Thy tired body will rest and heal

Friends are ever near

Ye are love

Your body aches

Release your pain

Waste not your energy on false fears

Love comes with compassion

Know this . . . it is true

All is revealed

In the present moment

Leading to trust and love

Heaven calls to you with great love

Release all fears unto the light

Embrace the shadow

Giving thanks for wisdom received

Wisdom leads to new heights of being

Deep inside of you know the truth of the Heart
of Hearts

Angels sing for you

Feel healing energies moving through your
body
Feel the joy of knowing "All is well"

Your path straightens to new adventures
Unknown -- yet known
Old -- yet new

Walk up the crystal staircase

    Embrace your blessings with gratitude

       Begin the journey

You cannot seek what is not meant to be

    So follow your heart, your soul

    Remembering --

      Respect yourself

        Love yourself

          Give yourself

Sensitivity lies in the heart of giving

'Tis easy to fear

To hide behind thy face

Not to venture forth

Not to find new horizons

> Keep up the walls
>
> Build armies of might
>
> Fear all those you near
>
> 'Tis easy to fear

Yet to open thy self to all that is anew

Unknown paths, unknown faces

'Tis growth of life

Not easy to face

As changes ye must make

> Yet, where fear has left
>
> Only happiness and love remain

Listen to your heart

You will know the way

The truth of God is in each moment

Where love is shared in tenderness

A unity of thoughts and dreams

As the light glows from within the soul
Feel its ever presence

Its warmth, love and hope shining forth to
guide

To show the way of faith, of eternity
To bring forth the message of love

For all who seek

Still is your heart as the morning dew

Rises to the sun with joy

The breath of sunshine

Opens your heart to love

Dwell not in the past

You are safe, loved

The spiral swirls quickly now

Waves of love and laughter fill the air

Feel the embrace of angels

Hear their tunes resounding

Dance to the flute

Sing your songs of joy

Filling your thoughts with love

In your heart, you hold the key
To your love and success

Be ever true to your truth
Ever loving with yourself

It is true the path seems rough but ye
Soar through shadows reaching heights unknown

Living in truth and grace
Giving to those in need

Sharing abundance with love and laughter

It is time to feed your soul with love and healing

Kindness from within

-- Peaceful moments of sharing

-- Peaceful moments of listening

-- Peaceful moments of being

It is springtime for you

The lilacs' sweetness fills the chapel

A melody plays on

Seraphim sing to you

    Of Harmony,

        Peace,

           Love,

                A Oneness with God

You walk the pathway of the stones

To a clearing in the forest

Deep in the forest lies a crystal stone

Hold it in your hand feeling its warmth

Open and let the light burst forth

For all to see, to share, to love

All future joys are now

Immerse in the light

Enjoy yourself

   Soar, soar, soar

Energy abounds

Flow with the tides of heaven

To the unknown, to success

The four winds have blown ye to a place of

Understanding

Live in that truth

The breath of sunshine

The freshness of the new fallen snow

Brings joy to your heart nourishing your soul

The unsung bird

Soon to sing its song

Soon to soar the mighty skies

Unfilled dreams appear with ease

Climb to the mountain's top

Only there is freedom to be

Free to love in unknown splendour

Soar the mighty skies

The gilded wings enwrap you

From the mountain you soar as one

The journey home begins

Higher and higher Eagle flies

        Glistening wings, radiant light

The valley below so lush and green

        Bursting buds, crocus in bloom

The awakening heart

        Bringing sweet love everlasting

Still is your heart as the morning dew

        Rises to the sun with joy

Call to the heavens of love

        Open to the new embrace

The Saints of old call to ye

   Ye are your own judge

      Ye choose your own path

         Ye create your every thought

The Keeper of the door calls to you

   Not to abandon the trail

      Keep strong within your truth

         Your love conquers all

         Reveals all

The Heart of Hearts shines upon thee

Savor the loving essences that surround you

Loving you, protecting you

Unseen by many, yet alive and vibrant

Believe,

Ask,

You will receive

Still is your mind

Open is your heart

It is not anywhere, not anyone

It is lightness, love of Self

To radiate your love to others

To share your joy every moment

To be one in love

With All

With open heart,

    Passion of the soul ignites

Within a circle, spirals whirling to the light

In the light thou doth join, a melding, a

oneness

    A beginning . . .

Part II

A Daily Guide for Meditation and Self-reflection

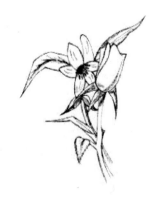

From the Garden Within

A Daily Guide for Meditation
and Self-reflection

For years I have owned an old book, containing daily inspirational thoughts by Longfellow called *Roses and Lilies*, printed in Boston in 1896. When roses and lilies grew in my garden a few years ago without my planting them, I knew they were a special message for me. Roses have always represented love to me and lilies have been a symbol of purity and union with the Divine. I began to write this part and *Messages from the Garden Within* based on my meditations. I hope to inspire the belief that each day is a beginning, a time to refresh, to flourish with new thoughts and to make changes to enrich your life. Meditation is the pathway to your garden within where your inner consciousness, your soul, dwells in peace. Open your garden gate and take a step forward on your spiritual journey to discover your messages within your soul.

When I first began to use meditation to relieve stress, and to relax, I discovered a deeper, intimate connection to God that felt amazing. I no longer was alone! I started to marvel at my spiritual experiences as I slowly began to trust in a loving universal source. In silence, I would go within to a place of quiet where the garden gate would open and lead me to wonderful visions and new thoughts that were awesome and beyond description.

Meditation is an experience, a personal journey within your mind, heart, and soul that leads to a greater understanding of your daily challenges and events. To be healthy and happy, you need a balance between the mind (your ego or personality), the body (your physical being) and the soul (your spiritual being). Meditation provides a connection for your outer world to meet your inner world and eases this union so you see life through new perceptions. As the mind becomes quiet, you become more receptive and more open to creative ideas and compassionate feelings. You begin to view life's unsettling events, as part of your journey and part of your learning, that lead you to a more positive point of view. With a shift in perspective, you have greater confidence and, most importantly, you have a better understanding of your beliefs, of your values and of who you really are. To transform to higher levels of consciousness and understanding requires that you discard many of your old beliefs, old fears and anxieties that weigh you down when you are meant to fly!

Anyone, from children to the aged, can meditate and enjoy its benefits. As a daily practice, meditation helps calm and relax your body so you can view life in a positive well-balanced manner. Scientific studies show that stress caused by everyday fears, anxieties and anger makes our bodies ill. As your body releases tensions, it begins to heal itself and return to a state of good health. Meditation allows you to release negative thoughts and energies leaving you with a clearer focus and sense of well-being.

Something wonderful happens as you meditate over time. Your mind begins to open to a new awareness as you begin to trust the inner voice you hear, to remember the symbols and colours that you visualize, and to use your intuitive abilities. It refreshes your memory and stimulates your inner consciousness. With greater inner consciousness, you experience greater connection with others, with universal energies and with the Divine Source. Meditation is about making a spiritual connection with the Divine Source that is beyond our daily illusions or realities. If you allow yourself greater spiritual connections, you will also learn to trust and allow things to develop and bloom in mysterious and wonderful ways.

It is in the seeking of your spiritual connection that you discover another dimension or place within your consciousness where there are no fears or anxieties. In reaching this inner place, you experience true peace and stillness. Knowing that this place of peace exists within brings comfort as you begin to see the true essence of your soul. Now, you begin to experience each day with new perceptions. You see purpose in each shadow and in each joy. Your life becomes fuller and richer as you feel and sense everything vividly. Your body feels more energized and alive. With this increased energy comes the need to stay balanced and focused in all you do. Creative visualization and meditation are wonderful tools for keeping our body, mind and spirit well balanced.

I begin my meditations with a short ritual by lighting a candle, playing soft music, chanting or playing my drum. I burn white sage or incense to cleanse the energies around me. I offer a prayer of thanksgiving for all my blessings. Rituals are meaningful and help connect us to our spiritual guides in the Divine Order of the Universe. Each religion has meaningful rituals that it integrates into religious services. You will be able to develop your own rituals or use some from your religion. They will help you to create a sacred space as you begin your meditation.

Twelve Easy Steps for Meditation

1. Meditation can only begin when you are able to concentrate with no distraction. Give yourself permission to have some quiet time each day. Most people begin meditating for ten to fifteen minutes a day. Find a place where you feel comfortable. You may like to sit on the floor or carpet, or in a chair, stretch out on a sofa, or sit outside under a tree. Find a place where you feel comfortable and will not be disturbed.

2. To meditate you need to be in a relaxed state. I have an imaginary shelf where I store my problems before I meditate. If negative thoughts push into your mind, do not give them permission to be there. However, do not strain or force your mind to concentrate. Just be still and relax. Read

the thought of the day from the following *Messages from the Garden Within*. Take a few minutes to focus on those words and contemplate the message. Then release all attachment to these words and visions. Let them go.

3. Close your eyes and allow your mind to be still. Begin by breathing in through your nose, holding your breath for a few seconds and exhaling through your mouth. Breathe gently as you concentrate on your breathing. Feel your body becoming more and more relaxed. Focus on your breathing. As you inhale think "I am," and as you exhale think "relaxed." Feel the rhythm of your body.

4. As you relax, connect with your body and check for any tension. If your feet feel tired and tense, flex your toes and relax them. Do the same with your legs, torso, arms, neck, shoulders and face. Breathe in as you flex; breathe out as you relax. Think, "I am relaxed." Imagine your breath reaching right down to the soles of your feet and connecting with Mother Earth. Feel your body relaxing. Breathe into any part that is tense or sore. Feel your body filling with warm energy that is soothing and calming.

5. Now, gently concentrate on the spot on your forehead between your eyebrows. This is the chakra, or energy center, that opens your intuition. By concentrating on this spot, it helps you to stay in the moment. If your mind wanders, bring your awareness back to this spot or to your breathing.

6. Above your head, imagine a beautiful, golden light. Feel its loving rays shining down and through you. Bring in this Divine, universal light energy into your heart space. Surrender and trust in the Divine Spirit as you experience your heart filling up with thoughts of love and peace. Feel this love increasing until it fills your heart space. It begins overflowing into your body and caressing every cell. Embrace this loving, healing energy. Only the most Divine energies are in your place of silence as you meditate. Breathe gently and enjoy the quiet stillness within. The Divine Spirit is within you.

7. In this quiet state, you can visualize whatever you want. Go to your favourite garden, seashore, mountain or think of the thought for the day. Continue to feel your body and muscles relaxing and feeling lighter and lighter.

8. During meditation, you can take a few moments to visualize your future the way you want it to be. See all the prosperity and good health, the career and activities that you desire in your life. Feel happy, refreshed and energized from all this abundance. Give thanks for your future blessings and for the many blessings you have already received. From a place of gratitude, we manifest our thoughts and dreams.

9. Now, take some time to listen and relax in silence. Enjoy the quiet and deep peaceful place you are sensing. You may see colours, symbols, light or even experience sounds and fragrances. Just enjoy the moment. Take a deep breath in and say "Ahhhhh" as you exhale ... feel the peace within.

10. This is the time when you may also call on your angels or spirit guides (according to your religious beliefs) to assist you. If you need guidance in any area of your life, simply ask for the best way to proceed for your highest good. You may hear an answer immediately or you may receive a message in a different way during the next few days. Give thanks for this assistance. Know you are always loved and protected and are never alone.

11. When you are ready, slowly bring your thoughts back into your space and open your eyes. Do not rush yourself. Take time to reflect about your feelings, visions or sounds that you received during your meditation. Feel the love within. Feel the joy within. Feel the gentle peace within.

12. Allow a few more minutes of quiet time to write your thoughts in a daily journal. Some people like to use this time to write poetry, songs or create artwork. It is amazing how creativity flows after meditation. You will soon be building a collection of your own creative ideas and messages. Do not question what you hear. I have found that even though I may not have understood a message at the time, later the meaning may appear in my daily life through books, the media, family, friends or even strangers. Often, through another meditation, I understand the message with greater depth and clarity.

Combining visualization with meditation is a powerful tool that I use towards manifesting my desires. Each day, I exactly visualize all my desires and my life full of abundance and joy. I have always treasured my two paintings of Native American children, a baby girl and a young boy. I received them as a gift years before we adopted our son Andrew and our daughter Sarah who are native Mayans from Guatemala. One day I held Andrew's first school photograph next to my painting of the young native boy. There was Andrew in both pictures! It was as if the artist had painted a picture from his school photo. I realized that I had been visualizing Andrew for years through this picture. The baby girl picture was similar to my daughter Sarah. Both children had manifested in my life and made my dream of being a mother come true. My children came to me at the right time in my life, and my visualizations came true.

You can manifest your desires by creative visualization and by feeling the passion of your desires before they happen. Be specific about your desires. Let these images be part of your daily meditations. If you need some healing, visualize your body being healthy during your meditation. Meditation does not replace medical care, but may enhance it. Remember how you felt when you were healthy and bring that feeling into the present moment. Recall a time when you were most happy and take a few minutes to enjoy that memory. Then bring that feeling of happiness into the present moment. Begin to feel the joy and well-being you desire. We truly are what we think and feel, so begin today by thinking only positive thoughts. Visualize your life exactly how you would like it to be with abundance, good health and joy!

During meditation you enter a sacred place where you remember who you are and what you value and enjoy. If you are just beginning to experience meditation, do not have expectations of some great awakening or spiritual vision. Allow yourself the opportunity to achieve deep relaxation and to get to know your inner Self. View it as you would a new budding friendship or relationship. Be most gentle and kind with yourself. Over time, you will be able to meditate for longer periods. There are many forms of meditation. One of my favourite meditations is a walking meditation where I go outside and deeply connect with everything around me. Sometimes I do a movement meditation where I put on soothing music and dance with it or I sit with my drum and relax with the gentle beats. I love group meditations in my workshops and seminars, as we all receive the loving energy that the group is creating. However, my deepest meditations are when I am in a quiet place alone in silence.

In the following *Messages from the Garden Within*, there is a daily thought suggesting an action and a prose for your meditation. Let your mind relax and open to expand the wonderful thoughts. Begin to feel love and peace within as you reflect upon the *Messages from the Garden Within*. Meditate on these reflections for greater understanding and wisdom to nourish your inner garden. May your meditations help you move gently towards greater self-awareness and happiness.

Messages from the Garden Within

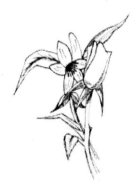

Enter the garden of love
Grow in the light of beauty
As the vision comes to lead you
On the garden path towards the whole
To the peace dwelling deep within

A Daily Guide for Meditation and Self-reflection

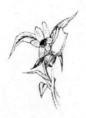

First Day

Create a day of Change

Be open and aware

See life as an adventure a journey

Into oneness into love

Into joy

Enjoy the unfolding mystery

A Daily Guide for Meditation and Self-reflection

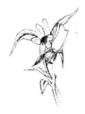

Second Day

Enjoy a day of Surprises

Energy abounds

Flow with the tides of heaven

Open to new explorations

Listen to Mourning Dove's call

Knowing the beauty and joy of the unknown

A Daily Guide for Meditation and Self-reflection

Third Day

Awaken to a day of Renewal

Rise up to the stars to the morning sun

Awaken to rebirth, to a life anew

Unknown, yet known

Old, yet new

Rejoice!

A Daily Guide for Meditation and Self-reflection

Fourth Day

Be calm on this day of Wonderment

Revel with the joys of spring, the spring of your life

Where love abides, truth abides

Be alive . . .

Willing . . .

Trusting . . .

A Daily Guide for Meditation and Self-reflection

Fifth Day

Frolic on this day of Merriment

Hear the sounds of the universe

So joyous are the tunes

So loving are the words

Let laughter fill your soul

Sing, sing, sing

Dance, dance, dance

A Daily Guide for Meditation and Self-reflection

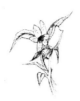

Sixth Day

Embrace this day of Strength

Venturing into truth,

A sense of security leads

To an inner sense of strength

Of hope

Become a spiritual warrior

Of love

A Daily Guide for Meditation and Self-reflection

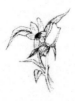

Seventh Day

In silence greet this day of Listening

Still is your heart

As the dawn greets you

Open your ever-questing mind

Listen to thy heart self

Love is the eternal answer

A Daily Guide for Meditation and Self-reflection

Eighth Day

Honour all life on this day of Respect

Honouring the right to be

You in all your splendour

Your love radiating

Compassion for all

As your gentleness touches

Those in need

A Daily Guide for Meditation and Self-reflection

Ninth Day

Rise to a day of Clearing

Free your heart of unwanted chains

Truly release with everlasting forgiveness

The torch burns ever within

The eternal flame rises to new heights

The heart releases, refills, renews

A Daily Guide for Meditation and Self-reflection

T enth Day

Smile on this day of Enjoyment

Deep in your soul a calling rings
Now is the moment

To reveal, to create, to shine
In all your beauty
Satisfaction comes from true passion
True passion brings joyous harmony

A Daily Guide for Meditation and Self-reflection

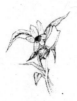

Eleventh Day

Rejoice in a day of Celebration

Whistling through the tall pines

The four winds howl with cheer

Whispering their song in your ear

The harps play out as dancers twirl

The trumpets sound as angels sing

"All is well"

"All is well"

A Daily Guide for Meditation and Self-reflection

Twelfth Day

Become enlightened on this day of Vision

A warming of your heart

A dream of tomorrow

With hopes of yesterday

Ever present in today

Go beyond the tomorrows

To new horizon

See the light of day

A Daily Guide for Meditation and Self-reflection

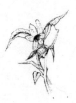

Thirteenth Day

Trust on this day of Knowing

Believe and you will receive

Healing rays of love

To those who ask

A simple task

A simple faith of love

Heaven's blessings are endless

Unlimited, omnipresent

A Daily Guide for Meditation and Self-reflection

Fourteenth Day

Breathe gently on this day of Transformation

In your silence is your knowing

With changing perception comes a new view

Transforming, blossoming with tenderness

Filled with creative thoughts within your sacred space

Emerging as abundant success and joy

A Daily Guide for Meditation and Self-reflection

Fifteenth Day

Gently embrace yourself on this day of Forgiving

Only in love is there light

All else fails

Conflict rises from lack of love

Love expands all thoughts

Compassion for all

Forgiveness heals, restores love

In new dimensions with sincerity

With honesty

A Daily Guide for Meditation and Self-reflection

Sixteenth Day

Sincerity fills this day of Prayer

Angels in the sky

Ever so near

Come to my side

Abide with me

Protect and shine

Through me

To see the light

Of truth and love

In deepest gratitude

For the loving source

Of my abundance

A Daily Guide for Meditation and Self-reflection

Seventeenth Day

Open to a day of great Awareness

You are on a path of righteousness

Take heed of all learning

Of all you survey

Feel for those in need

Trust in the process

Ever is a light of understanding

A Daily Guide for Meditation and Self-reflection

Eighteenth Day

Soar on this day of Freedom

The silver bird flies high with gilded wings

Sparkling like diamonds

Bringing renewal and revelation

Rejoice and spread the breathless beauty

Embrace the freedom within

Moments of true bliss

Soar   Soar   Soar

A Daily Guide for Meditation and Self-reflection

Nineteenth Day

Immerse in this day of Remembrance

Listen to the words of the ancient ones

Keep the faith of yesteryear

Dwell in this moment

The time is yours to live and explore

A remembrance of all your power

And love for all

A Daily Guide for Meditation and Self-reflection

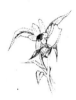

Twentieth Day

Walk softly on this day of Tenderness

Tenderness soothes your soul

Heals your heart space

Bringing loving thoughts to you

Your beauty, your tenderness

Your awareness

Reflecting your caring soul

Awakening to the oneness

Feeling the connection

To all creation

A Daily Guide for Meditation and Self-reflection

T wenty-first Day

Be thankful on this day of Understanding

In your heart, you hear the ancient ones

It goes beyond the ages to the King of Kings

The united love of the universe

You swing from the golden cords

Ever united, ever one

A Daily Guide for Meditation and Self-reflection

Twenty-second Day

Marvel on this day at life's Mystery

You cannot seek what is not to be

So follow your heart, your soul

Fear not the forward journey

A bud takes warmth

Gentle spring rains

Watch the mystery of nature

How awesome in its beauty

A Daily Guide for Meditation and Self-reflection

Twenty-third Day

Feel joyous on this day of Happiness

Laughter brings you perspective

In times of deepest shadows

Mending your aching heart

Changing each moment into joy

Smile, you deserve it

A Daily Guide for Meditation and Self-reflection

T wenty-fourth Day

Flow with ease on this day in Dreamtime

Embark on your spiritual journey

Let your spirit soar flying without wings

Amongst the heavens of sparkling lights

Brilliant colours in whirling spirals

With the light of love beaming

Knowing all is beautiful

In this timeless moment

A Daily Guide for Meditation and Self-reflection

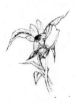

Twenty-fifth Day

Recall your essence on this day of Youthfulness

Sifting through the sands of time

Memories of beings, visions of souls

Your thoughts clear now with new learning

Delve into your being

To the fountain of youth ever present

Find your inner child and embrace

Play, laugh in the bright sunshine

With your companion in love

A Daily Guide for Meditation and Self-reflection

Twenty-sixth Day

Work diligently on this day of Learning

If you choose to repeat a lesson

It will come again

Truly release all anger and fears

With loving forgiveness

Then and only then does the repetition end

The path widens to new awareness

But keep on track

Seek the highest good for all

In all your thoughts and deeds

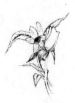

T wenty-seventh Day

Feel the loving embrace of Friendship

In your deepest being, you know the truth

Love will endure the test of time

Once again a union, a friendship of ages

Once again a love, undefined

With the freedom to simply be

Opening fully to its greatest beauty

A Daily Guide for Meditation and Self-reflection

T wenty-eighth Day

Play on this day of Well-Being

Dance with the dolphins

Among the foamy waves

Emerge

With the breath of life

The joy of play

Singing your songs of old

Become in tune with their vibrations

Lifting you to greater heights

A Daily Guide for Meditation and Self-reflection

Twenty-ninth Day

Heal on this day of Trusting

React not to another's fears

Stay centered in your Self

You are on the path of righteousness

Take the route of least resistance

Time of preparation

Time of commitment

Open your heart in triumph

See gifts on a silver tray

Trust what you see

Share with those who seek to know

A Daily Guide for Meditation and Self-reflection

Thirtieth Day

Receive on this day the gift of Love

Like a beautiful rose love unfolds

Nothing to seek

It is all there

Feelings of truth and love

Leading to the union of hearts

As you journey home to oneness

Together

A Daily Guide for Meditation and Self-reflection

Thirty-first Day

Experience this day as a Beginning

From a decision comes a commitment

From a commitment comes a trust

From a trust -- the universe responds

Evolving with bountiful joy

Surrender . . . trust . . . love . . .

The universe will radiate blessings to you

Part III

Nature's Guide to Spiritual Awareness

The Gates of Wisdom open with a caring heart
Grow in the light of nature's beauty

Listen with your heart self
Fly with endless freedom

Nature's Guide to Spiritual Awareness

In our expanding knowledge, power and highly-developed technology, we have forgotten some basic truths and wisdoms. We see these truths, passed down to us through ages by religions and cultures, each day in nature. All animals, plants and minerals are my life's teachers who bring deep understandings and assist my remembrance of who I am. They have assisted me to learn about life's mysteries. The *Messages of Wisdom* come from my experiences with nature's teachers and I share with you some of the lessons I have experienced. The interpretation of the teachings is from my experience and is not from a specific Native American or aboriginal tribe. Some teachings may be similar to Native American beliefs. Aboriginal peoples have long sought and learned lessons from their environment, from the howling of the four winds, from a babbling brook, from the call of the loon, or from the web of the spider. Each tribe has various teachings of the meanings and symbols of nature's teachers. One tribe may have one meaning for a fish while another tribe may have found a different meaning for the same fish. It is important to become open to the spiritual teachings from many sources. The more connected I am to my environment with all its beauty and teachings, the more wisdom I discover. It is all there. All I have to do is stop, look and listen.

Many symbols have come to be significant in my meditations. I encourage you to seek your own meanings of symbols that repeat and reflect the true meanings of your existence and your truth, those that define your true self. As I tap into symbols in nature, I often find humour while I watch animals and birds, and discover beauty and peace in plants, flowers and trees. These symbols give my life greater depth and meaning by revealing spiritual attributes.

Begin by becoming aware of the animals, insects, and plants that you are attracting. It may feel uncomfortable at first, but talk to your plants, to your birds in the garden or the squirrel in the tree. Scientists tell us that everything is energy, vibrating energy and each plant is vibrating energy and responds to energy around it. Your voice or soft music will soothe your plant and encourage its growth because it feels your loving energy and it will respond to it. Because we all are energy beings, we are interdependent with one another. It is when each of us develops compassion and caring for all beings that the healing of humanity and of our planet begins.

From my relationships with different animals, plants and insects, I have associated each message in my *Messages of Wisdom*. For example, I returned to university when I was forty years old. I was recently divorced, alone and scared, but each morning I would see the seagulls soaring high in the sky outside my window. As I drove to university, I would still see them flying overhead and I began to sense that they were signs of hope. Uncle Howard loved seagulls because he saw them as survivors. I remembered his teachings when I saw the gulls and since then the seagull became my symbol of hope. Over the years, other significant messages came from nature. The maple, pine, and tamarack trees became friends, as did the roses, pansies and water lilies. Each plant or animal helped to create a thought to remind me of the very lesson or the spiritual attribute that would help me at that moment.

I began to share my experiences with my friends only to discover that they too received messages. In fact, my family members and friends have similar teachers in nature. My friends, Barbara and Dee, have crows near them, while Sharon has Canada geese near her as she walks her dog in the fields. Margaret has her backyard rabbit and mourning dove who visit regularly. Aunt Beverley loves lilacs, as I do. My husband Ian admires our backyard maple tree, known as "Alfie," that has marvelous beauty for us to embrace. Andrew has a great affinity for the tiger, and Sarah collects rocks and enjoys seeing shapes in the clouds. Our family dog, Ginger, a lively Shih-Poo, energizes us everyday with her whimsical playfulness. My Mom, Dad and brother Bob loved the call of the loons at our summer cottage on Lake Penache in northern Ontario. Aunt Genevieve taught me to connect with the stars that are so vivid on summer evenings.

Everyone can find solace from his or her surroundings in the darkest of times. There is always beauty in nature to uplift us and help us to transform. There is always light beyond our shadows. It is in the desire of more understanding and joy in our life that we find the most help from nature. How can one not be in awe of a budding rose, or the transformation of a caterpillar into a butterfly or the uniqueness of each delicate snowflake? It is truly beyond our comprehension. However, we do not have to understand life as it is the great mystery. Our task is simply to enjoy and experience life to our fullest by developing our talents, skills and sharing them with others. Most of us are too busy to take time to feel good and we become ill as our lives become unbalanced. Observe the symmetry in nature. Through this balance, we can share this planet with ease and companionship with all beings. Look to see how humans are destroying this balance, and think of what you can do each day to protect our environment so our children can grow up with earth under their feet, instead of concrete.

Can you see yourself as a guardian of the earth who assists in its healing and its peacemaking? I know I often get so involved in my family and personal life that I disconnect from what is happening in the world events. Perhaps, it is because listening about wars and our deteriorating planet is too painful. Yet, I know that I cannot hide away and deny my connection to all life. I am responsible for what happens in this world. I can make a difference each day and so can you. Let us make our world a greener and more balanced place to live. You may wonder what you can do to assist our planet and humanity. Here are some simple, powerful steps.

How to Assist our Planet and Humanity

- Visualize each day how you would like your world to be.

- Put all your energy into positive good thoughts and let negative thoughts fall away. Positive thoughts attract positive happenings and positive energies. Your thoughts and actions are important to all of us.

- Feel your peace within and know that this is the truth.

- Extend that peace to all you meet by viewing each person, plant and animal as a Beloved one who deeply connects with you.

- Send thoughts, prayers of love and peace to all by expanding your prayers to include everything on our planet.

Remember your feelings create your manifestations. As you integrate into your life the actions that will assist all humanity, you will begin to feel a beautiful connection to all, a natural connection that blossoms and expands through love. All over this planet, people are awakening to a renewed sense of love . . . to the power and essence of love. Let your messages of wisdom from nature come into your life, as you move deeply into your truth and love. It is with great honour and respect for nature's teachers that I share with you some of the teachings I have received. Each page in *Messages of Wisdom* has a word of wisdom, a prose and the lesson. Quiet your mind before opening the following part of this book. Let the book fall open to a page and use the animal or plant message to awaken thoughts in you during your meditation. Does its message resonate with you? Does it have some guidance for you, today? If it does, keep this animal or plant in your mind as you meditate. After you meditate, write down any thoughts you may have received that expand the message.

Developing your own message sharpens your intuition and you will begin to trust your intuition, your innate gift of knowing within your Sacred Heart. Some call it our "sixth" sense. I call it my "soul sense" as I feel my intuition is a direct link to universal consciousness and guidance. It takes time to trust your intuition, but it is always available to you. Intuition is a natural feeling, so you will feel comfortable as your Sacred Heart guides you.

We can experience our intuition in many ways:

- A feeling about something that occurs without any effort
- A feeling that alerts you to pay attention
- A sense of something as your stomach flutters
- A chills runs up your arms or body
- An "ah ha" feeling, this is intuition kicking in
- A vision or premonition about the future
- An inner voice that protects and guides
- A feeling telling you something is right or wrong
- A feeling that you can trust
- A vision in meditation
- A symbol in nature

Intuition guides us by showing what is best for us in this moment. I want to live in the now, to create in the now, and to live in the present moment and let the future manifest from my present feelings. You can use your intuition to increase your understanding of the symbols in nature that you encounter daily. As you connect with nature, your intuition will clarify the meanings of messages from animals, insects and plants. They may be similar to mine or they may have a completely different message for you.

Most of all have fun and enjoy your time in nature. Sing with the cardinals. Bark with the dogs. Waddle with the ducks! Smile at your plants. Awaken to the bountiful gifts and teachings of nature. Awaken all of your senses to discover how wonderful you are!

Your life is full of blessings, joys and deep peace
In nature, open your Sacred Heart to discover
Love,
Joy,
Oneness
Wonderful beginnings, creativity and success greet you
on your spiritual journey
All is Well

Messages of Wisdom

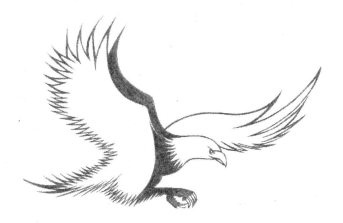

From Nature's Teachers

The Wisdom of EAGLE

Observe

Soar, soar, soar

To the highest mountain top

and beyond

Soar, soar, soar

To heighten awareness

With new perceptions

Soar, soar, soar

With the Spirit and

Love of timelessness

Seek to rise above difficult shadows by becoming an observer of yourself. Be non-judgemental, non-critical, and always self-loving. Soar with Eagle to greater knowing and learning of the Universe. Feel free in spirit to fly with ease. Rise above and observe your world with clearness, sharpness, fearlessness.

The Wisdom of ROSE

Love

The fragrances of roses

Bring sweet memories

Of you

Walking side by side

Hand in hand

In love

Like a beautiful rose, love blooms. You do not have to seek love because you are love. Within your heart is a source of unconditional love. Feel the essence of your love and let it grow, expand it and send it to those whom you love. Now increase your love again, ever expanding it so it touches all you meet and beyond. In truth, there is only love. Love is eternal.

The Wisdom of LILIES

Union

Feel the oneness you are

As the lilies gently sway

The garden gate opens

To a new world awaiting

Sharing love in tenderness

A unity of thoughts and dreams

Emerging as one beautiful love

As you develop a greater sense of Self, a greater remembrance of who you are, begin to feel a wonderful union with all life. Your sense of loneliness and separation will disappear. Feel your connection to all beings, all nature, to the universe. You are part and one with a loving source. You are on your pathway home to Oneness.

The Wisdom of BEAR

Transformation

From your silent cave

New thoughts arise

With changing perception

Comes transformation

To transform you must be a willing participant who takes time to work with your subconscious to take away your fears. Go into your cave, be silent, releasing all fears, emerging with a new positive view.

The Wisdom of BEAVER

Commitment

A builder in endless time

A worker of the heart

Whose commitment and persistence

Bring success

Make a decision and a commitment to your goal. Let your intention be heart centered. Then let the universal energies go to work for you. Trust always in the process. Miracles will happen!

The Wisdom of BUFFALO

Prayer

Though the pounding of your hoofs is gone

Your mighty spirit roams

Courageously across the plains

Bringing ancient messages

Through hope and prayer

The ancient wisdom is yours to discover. Listen to your inner soul, your inner wisdom. Ask for help through prayers in deepest gratitude. There is always hope as there is always an answer to your question. Ask, listen, and allow.

The Wisdom of BUTTERFLY

Patience

Coming from the dark into the light

Oh, Butterfly how wondrous

You survived life changes

With grace and beauty

What a true example of the miracles of Mother Nature! See the power in patience, in stillness and in growth. Look for beauty in all creatures, the grace in their being, the love in their hearts. Move through your transitions without resistance moving ever towards wholeness.

The Wisdom of COYOTE

Laughter

There are many tricks

Many jokes, many fools

Yet, from each

A lesson is learned

Laugh with Coyote

Live to the fullest

The joker is ever near. Learn to laugh at life's absurdities. Lighten up! Do not take yourself and others so seriously. Walk softly, dance lightly, and laugh heartily. Watch for Coyote. He is a teaser.

The Wisdom of DOLPHIN

Harmony

Call of the Dolphin

A song of the sea

Creating perfect harmony

Love, peace and freedom

For all who seek

Think of how your life would be if it were truly harmonious. What changes can you make to increase harmony in all aspects of your life? Remember how it feels to be healthy and strong. Remember to breathe the energies of the universe into your body to heal gently each day. Feel good and enjoy the freedom of being you.

The Wisdom of DOG

Loyalty

In your silence

In your playfulness

You are here

Ever faithful, ever loyal

Companion of my heart

A friend is a person who knows your deepest shadows and weaknesses, but only sees your beauty. A loyal friend loves you because you are you. Know that each person's soul is an essence of love. Become one with that love.

The Wisdom of RABBIT

Shadow

Explore the unknown

Fear not the present shadows

Let the four winds blow you

To a place of understanding

Where fear has left

Only happiness remains

Live in that truth

Your fears that linger in the shadow are your greatest inhibitors. They are illusions. They are not real. They are simply "what ifs," but if you give energy to this negativity, you will attract exactly what you are feeling. Conversely, your positive feelings and affirmations attract good energies.

The Wisdom of FROG

Creativity

Sing your heart song with me

Leap through the air

Become the breath of spirit

Let all possibilities be

Our thoughts and feelings create all our actions. Let your creative juices arise and create the life you have always wanted. Leap across the pond like a frog. Take a giant leap forward. Stay open to all opportunities. Allow yourself to blossom and share your creations.

The Wisdom of BLUE HERON

Renewal

Still, ever so still in the greenness
You stand at the edge of the pond
Hardly visible beside the tall bushes
How tall and elegant are you
Moving swiftly to catch your daily feed
Returning to your solitary stance

In stillness, ready yourself for rebirth of your soul, a renewal of spirit through your connection to the Divine Spirit. From within, truth lives. Listen. Creativity flourishes as new thoughts and feelings become activated.

The Wisdom of DEER

Tenderness

Your tenderness soothes my soul

Heals my heart

Bringing loving thoughts of you

Your beauty, your gentleness

Reflecting your caring soul

Beauty in motion

Across the open field

Awakening to the oneness

Of nature and spirit

Heal yourself with kindness, with tenderness, with love. Let your actions be gentle. Allow only those who come from a caring heart to enter your sacred space. Let loving energies emanate from you. Receive and give love to all.

The Wisdom of CROW

Ancient Ones

Crow tells of Ancient teachings

On tablets of stone

It is time of great gatherings, great awakenings

Heed the voice, the song of love

Share with joy your ancient days

Heed the call of the loving essences

Star of the Ancients leading you forth

The call of Crow awakens you to be aware of messages from within, from others, from nature. These messages come in words, sounds, or symbols and from our animal teachers. Tap into the universal consciousness to learn the ancient laws of the universe. Listen and grow in love. The Ancient Ones say the past does not have to be repeated, but the lessons remembered.

The Wisdom of CAT

Intuition

How quietly you watch the world
As you move through the garden
Walking gently through the ferns
With an inner knowing
A sense beyond to guide you

Open your heart space to greater intuitions. Develop this sense to become wiser, more sensitive and compassionate to the needs of others. Allow the loving·essences to guide you with their love. Open to the wisdom of your heart to trust your inner knowing.

The Wisdom of SQUIRREL

Trust

It comes to those who wait

Trusting in the process

Undying, unyielding universal love

Stretching forward courage

Embracing the challenge

Fearless, onward to success

Stay in the moment. Trust the universe wants you to have great success and will aid you every step of the way. Trust yourself. From trust, the universe opens your spiritual connections and life evolves with joy.

The Wisdom of WOLF

Teacher

Hear the haunting call of Wolf

Awakening thoughts of old

Teachings of transcendence

Uniting with the stars of heaven

Protector of the pack

Teacher of love and wisdom

Your teachers are ever near. They come and go during your lifetime, as you need them. You, like Wolf, are also a great teacher. Teach others to love through your radiance and forgiveness. Call for your teachers and they will assist you. Share you talents and skills to the fullest.

The Wisdom of SEAGULL

Hope

Stretching towards the dawn

Ever receptive to the light

Behind the drifting clouds

Crossing the bridge alone

Onward to new horizons

A view of a soaring gull

Whispering a call of hope

Hope is the motivation that encourages you to open the door of opportunity and take a step forward. It works hand-in-hand with faith and trust. There is always hope as you are always protected and loved. Let Seagull become a sign of this hope as it soars above you.

The Wisdom of SWAN

Dreamtime

In a pool of dreams

I see your reflection

The night sky glistens

With showers of light

An image of you appears

And I see love

We are spiritual beings experiencing a human existence. In waking or nighttime dreams, you can tap into a collective universal consciousness that is waiting for your awakening. Be a spiritual traveler and learn from your dreams.

The Wisdom of CARDINAL

Heart Love

The beauty of this day

Is magnified by the thought of you

Of your loving ways

Of your gentle voice

Singing a heart song

To my soul

The more you center yourself in love the more happiness you will experience. Come from a loving heart in all that you do. Be willing to love. Learn how to be more loving through acts of caring and kindness. If your daily happenings are going wrong, bring yourself back to your heart space. Center your thoughts in love, take a deep breath and allow love to radiate from you. Be open to receive love from others.

The Wisdom of HORSE

Courage

Walk carefully along the winding path

Head held high with eyes so clear

Feel the energy ever growing

Meet the windy fields with glee

Ride with courage into openness

Steadily moving, pounding hoofs

With lightning speed of a fearless spiritual warrior

of Divine love

Faith takes courage but as your knowing increases so does your courage. Have the courage to try something new or to do something you enjoyed as a child. Make the move and the Universe will help you and move with you. Ride with the winds and look ever forward to new adventures. Today you are a fearless warrior of love and compassion, of courage and strength.

The Wisdom of PANSY

Gentleness

You gently greet the spring

Days of rain, chilling nights

With grace and beauty

Opening to the morning rays

The warmth brings a smile

To your tender face

With a gentle thought, a gentle word, a gentle touch, love blooms. We often forget to be gentle with ourselves. Bathe yourself in nature's beauty. Smile at the flowers. Say hello to the wind. Listen to the songbirds. Be one with all. Feel the loving energies return to you. These friends are ever with you.

The Wisdom of LOON

Mystery

Keeper of the lake are ye

Surveyor of all

Your call echoes hauntingly

In the still of darkness

Telling of the mystery

So we may recall

As the snow gently covers the earth, it seems that all is dead. Yet beneath, the roots are alive. The unseen animals dwell in hibernation. Life continues even when unseen. The universal energies still exist but to many, they remain unseen. They, too, are alive and growing. Revel in life's unseen joys. Open your awareness to all possibilities.

The Wisdom of OWL

Silence

In your silence

Take flight

In your emptiness

Feel the harmony

In your awakening

Fill with light

In your knowing

Live your truth

In silence, seek your own truth, be discerning and trust you will receive what you need. Fear not others but fill with the loving light of the universe. Live in truth, honesty and peace.

The Wisdom of SALMON

Flow

The mighty river moves towards the sea

Rushing smoothly over the rocks

Bending swiftly with each turn

Always flowing, never yielding

To obstacles on its way home

Although Salmon travels against the stream, knowing its path is true, its intentions ever clear, it follows its pathway home. Allow your pathway to gently flow and bend without resistance, to guide you home to a place of peace and harmony.

The Wisdom of DOVE

Peace

The beauty of the Dove

So graceful and white

Hovers over you

Bringing peace and joy on its wings

In the stillness within peace dwells, creating a gentle embrace of love. In peace, you feel the presence of God, of oneness with all life. In peace, you become the Beloved and see the Beloved in each being. In peace, you are love.

Part IV

Creative Consciousness
Creating your Life

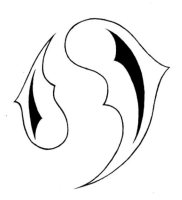

From your Inner Consciousness

Creative Consciousness
Creating your Life

One of the greatest benefits of meditation is that it helps develop your "creative consciousness," a consciousness where you are the co-creator of your life with the Divine Spirit. With a creative consciousness, you allow your creative expression to awaken in endless forms and something very mystical and spiritual begins to occur. You discover thoughts, ideas, art forms and sounds that seem to just spring from you. Artists often say that it is as if someone else is creating the picture, story or song. I know that feeling when I write after my meditations. I just allow the thoughts to enter my consciousness without effort, without questioning them. I always wonder at the "messages" that I receive. My pen moves over the page in scribbles and the words are always the words I need to hear. If I am not integrating them into my life, I hear the messages repeated, and I know that I needed to hear them again. I am truly thankful for these thoughts and ideas as they guide me through my life. I know the Divine Spirit loves me unconditionally and only speaks in words of love to me as my messages contain only beautiful thoughts about love, compassion, forgiveness and peace.

The greatest tool I have found to awaken my creativity is meditation. Meditation really is an art form, as I may see colours, forms, shapes with fascinating designs. Sometimes I hear intriguing sounds and chants that bring me comfort. They are like a new language with words such as "ta tee way tah." These celestial sounds are very soothing and nurturing. It is so amazing how they relax my body and mind. I often share these tunes with clients during a Natural Sound and Reiki session, a modality I offer for relaxation and energy balancing. Listen for new sounds during your meditations. Meditation will provide a personal, private artistic gallery just for you where you can explore your creative self and receive inspiration.

As you develop your creative consciousness, you come to an inner meeting with your Divine consciousness and your soul. You form a trust that each of your experiences, whether positive or negative from your perspective, occur to show you exactly what you need to learn or experience in each moment. As this trust expands so does your creativity as you begin to take steps to express your ideas or concepts, knowing they are part of your spiritual path. Yet, there is always the unknown with many unanswered questions that can still make us fearful. As you meditate and feel a Divine connection, you begin to sense that you are not alone on this human/spiritual journey. You connect in a mysterious, energetic way to spiritual beings for support and guidance. Your fears of the unknown begin to subside. So trusting in the unknown, embracing the unknown, and allowing the unknown to show peaceful living becomes your way of being. There is a shift in your perspective and a move towards experiencing your creative consciousness more fully.

The time is now to reveal your creative consciousness by using your inner talents in whatever way you desire to express your feelings, thoughts and inner knowing so we may all grow and benefit from your inner gifts. If you look back in history, you see artists and artisans who used their talents to express a glimpse of what they were experiencing in their lifetime. You do not have to be a great artist, but simply allow a way of self-expression to blossom and grow.

Your artistry, like the universe, is limitless and forever creating something new.

After many years of practicing meditation, it continues to bring me many benefits. It provides a place of silence, a sanctuary, where I experience a deep sense of peace. I have learned to use this space as a place to surrender my fears and anxieties to the Divine. I integrate my Christian beliefs through prayer and give thanks for my blessings. All of the major world religions teach meditation and prayer. During meditation, I begin to feel a union with the perfect presence of God. I receive an indescribable feeling of love and support through the images I receive, and through a deep knowing that I am somehow connected and part of a loving source that assists me to greater knowing of my Self. I know that I am a spiritual being, a being of universal light energy that unites all life. I am learning about my creative powers so I may create with my every thought and feeling! This knowing is so empowering and liberating! It allows me to embrace my personal will power and my Divine nature. My creative consciousness gives me freedom to be me. I am a co-creator of life with the Divine Spirit.

Be conscious of your true feelings, as it is easy to fool yourself or to be in denial. This honesty will assist you to take off your masks and reveal the authentic you. Love is a risk that requires vulnerability but its rewards are limitless, and astounding miracles occur. Love is the key to expanding your creative consciousness.

A Time for Peace

"In peace, you are love."

In 2004, I was ordained as a Minister of Spiritual Peacemaking by the Beloved Community founded by James Twyman, an internationally known Peace Troubadour. At that time I made a commitment to have peace in my life by saying *"YES, YES, YES"* to peace. Try saying these words. They are so powerful and grounding. Once I made this commitment, issues, that needed clearing in all areas of my life, started to rise up. When this clearing first happened, it was a little disconcerting, and I wondered if I could ever feel peaceful. Then I realized that I had many things to discard and a cleansing had to occur. Perhaps for some it is enough to say, "Yes, I want peace in my life," but I knew I had to take action steps to begin creating it and to being truly peaceful.

 Ten Action Steps for Peaceful Living

Step 1. Letting Go

"Letting go" is a giant step towards healing and peace. Many years ago, I started letting go of things that were not working for me on all levels . . . emotionally, mentally, spiritually, and physically. This meant that I had to change by releasing old patterns and old stuff. I had to find a "new way" of being. My "old way" was difficult to change. However, as I made positive changes, I evolved in many ways that moved me forward. Recently, Ian and I took a big step by letting go of our retail store. This action created new space in my life. I had time to be with my family, to create our new website, to expand my holistic services by becoming a Reiki Master/Practitioner, and to complete this book! I felt a new sense of freedom.

Many years ago when I was alone and preparing to be divorced, I had difficulty letting go of my past. I received a gift of wisdom from my friend Helen who shared some tips on the meaning of "letting go." They helped me a great deal with my process of releasing the past and moving ahead.

o *To let go is to forgive myself and to forgive others.*

o *To let go is not to regret the past, but to grow and live for the future.*

o *To let go is to fear less and love more.*

o *To let go is not to try to change or blame another, it is to make the most of myself.*

o *To let go is respecting another's right to choose.*

o *To let go is not to fix, but to be supportive.*

o *To let go is to stop trying to do it all by myself and to let God.*

o *To let go is to surrender to the will of God.*

Step 2. Opening to Heart Love

As you open your heart to love, you will feel this sense of freedom too. Others will see you changing as your inner light shines. Old patterns and energies that did not support you will fade away. Others will wonder what happened to create this change in you. Tell them you have found a new relationship with yourself and God that has opened your heart to love and peace within. Your love of God, of your Self, and of all life cannot be hidden as you are radiating it in every moment when you say, **"YES, YES, YES"** to peace in your life. This is when you truly surrender your fears and allow your life to manifest in a new way.

Step 3. Trusting

Can you believe that God knows what is best for you? Can you put your trust in God to show you a new way of living that will bring you the joy and love you deserve and desire? Think about a friend that you trust in your life and the qualities that person has. You may trust him/her because he/she understands you, forgives your errors and loves you unconditionally. Trust, understanding, forgiveness, and unconditional love are attributes of God. Your friend, whom you trust, is reflecting God's attribute of trust to you. You can trust God in every moment. Trusting is a huge step, but our fears stop us from this most important step. When you can feel the love and peace of the Divine presence within as you meditate, your fears begin to dissipate and your trust in Divine guidance begins to grow. Now, your body relaxes, your mind calms and your soul smiles.

Step 4. Allowing

Learning to listen is the key to allowing spiritual guidance to evolve. We can learn our best pathways by carefully listening to our meditations, our loved ones and friends; and to nature's messages. "Allowing" means we take off our blinders, open our eyes, and awaken our heart, to allow new events, people and thoughts to enter our life. Now we have multiple choices to make that can assist us to expand and evolve. Bring your awakened self fully into the present moment. Be open to receive without expectations, but with deepest joy and gratitude. God has created everything you need.

Step 5. Expressing Gratitude

In the midst of our busy lives, we often do not feel grateful for our life and all its gifts -- especially when stressed and ill or when life feels hopeless and sad. Everything is a gift to us to help us to awaken to God's unconditional love and the infinite beauty of the universe. Lighter energy surrounds you when you are grateful and by saying a simple "thank you," you can create a new perspective towards your life that will offer you the healing and comfort you need. Be grateful for all your experiences in your life as they provide opportunities for a personal, intimate relationship with God, a deeper knowing of love and feeling the presence of God in each moment. In gratitude, your heart opens to accept unconditional love. You move into a greater knowing of the Divine consciousness of one heart and universal truth.

Step 6. Knowing your Intentions

Everything that evolves comes from our intentions. Do you know your intentions in all areas of your life -- physically, emotionally, mentally, and spiritually? Are your intentions coming from your Sacred Heart? Are they love-centered or are your choices coming from your ego-based thinking? Are your motives fear-based? Your intentions activate the energy to manifest your desires. Natural health practitioners know how their intentions powerfully affect the healing process with their clients. The clients feel the loving intention and compassion of the practitioner and their energy responds to this love; then natural healing occurs. Love heals us as each of our cells responds to love. As our cells become healthy, they move fully into their natural state of love. Love is our natural state and being. Knowing your intention with all your actions is so important to your spiritual growth. The intention of sharing your love, in whatever you are doing, leads you to creating peace in your life and in the life of others.

Step 7. Feeling Peaceful

The universe works in a cycle of giving and receiving. So if you want love, give love. If you want money, give money. If you want peace, be peaceful. As you meditate, find your inner place of peace each day and expand that loving feeling into every cell of your body. Feel the gentle embrace of peace filling your heart and mind, and allow your actions to come from that energy. Even if you do not feel completely peaceful, *imagine* how you would feel if you were peaceful with *a peaceful heart, a quiet mind, a joyful life.* Feeling peaceful becomes a natural way of being, as you know, within, there is a sacred temple of peace, a place of your true existence called your Sacred Heart. Here you are peace, purity and wholeness.

Step 8. Taking Creative Action

When you make a commitment to a life of peace, it is time to take creative action. Taking creative action will become easier now as your fears diminish and your vision of peace provides clarity for you to move forward to have your dreams manifest. Your life may become easier when you decide to clear your living space by getting rid of old belongings, or you may feel it is time to contact an old friend whom you have not seen for awhile. You can take small creative actions that will make a huge difference in your life and you soon see wonderful results. Trust that as you move into great light and love, you will know what steps to take without trying hard to figure out what you should be doing. You simply begin to know what is best for you. This is a most exciting adventure as your life begins to sparkle, shine and transform.

Step 9. Giving Service

As you move into a place of peace, your compassion for others grows and you will want to serve by committing to assist others. You are now a visionary of global peace and consciousness. Ask how you can best serve humanity. You have many opportunities to assist your family, friends and community. A beautiful way is simply to see each person as worthy and deserving of all life's gifts and to see each as a Beloved. As all of your actions are full of love and compassion, your service naturally evolves from your passionate heart to enrich your life and the lives of others. You are now a spiritual peacemaker.

Step 10. Loving Life

The life of a spiritual peacemaker is not without challenges. However, you know that each moment is precious and exciting. As you grow and evolve, you experience life fully. You see that your actions are not just important to you, but to others, and to all humanity. You want to help make our world a different place in some way -- a peaceful place. You begin to take steps within your own life and family to bring peace. Loving life means loving all people and nature, and feeling their connectedness and radiance glowing within them. It is time to lighten up, to relax and to enjoy the life you are creating. Remember the Coyote's message. *"Learn to laugh at life's absurdities. Lighten up! Do not take yourself and others so seriously. Walk softly, dance lightly, and laugh heartily."*

The time for peace is *now*! Throughout the world, millions of people desire peace. A wonderful shift is happening that will create a world of love and compassion. This is the time for all of us to discover our peaceful path, our inner peace. The world needs each of us to make this transformation so we can create universal peace to form a global community of trust, sharing and understanding. Everyone deserves abundance, peace and freedom. We all have an active role in our daily lives to make a global community of peace a reality. This shift, predicted by the ancients, is happening *now*, in spite of the wars and conflicts that will end. The light of love always outshines darkness. You begin within your Sacred Heart space with reverence for all life, and spread your joy and peace to others in your daily life. Take the time, in silence, during your meditation, for an exciting exploration of your inner self, your soul, as you co-create your peaceful path with God. Your life will transform in abundant, peaceful and wondrous ways.

About Jane Rosalea Booth

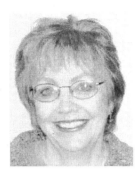

Jane is a Holistic Workshop Facilitator who created a program for holistic living and meditation called The Peaceful Path. Through her love of animals and nature, she found simple, yet profound messages for inner peace from nature's teachers. From her personal experiences, she discovered the power of creative visualization and meditation as keys to ancient wisdom, to self-awareness and intuition, and to inner spiritual strength for today's challenges.

For over 18 years, Jane has presented meditation and holistic workshops, in the Region of Waterloo, Ontario, to community and health organizations. In 2004, she became an Ordained Minister of Spiritual Peacemaking and received a Masters of Divinity. She holds a Bachelor of Arts in Social Development Studies and a Certificate of General Social Work. She is a Certified Sound Energy Dynamics Practitioner and Reiki Master. She is a former elementary school teacher. Jane lives with her family in Meaford, Ontario, where she hosts her business The Golden Light Centre for Well-Being Inc. Visit Jane at www.goldenlightcentre.com for her workshop and retreat schedules, peace projects, services and the Golden Light Wellness Shop. Visit www.in-silence.net her Official Author site. Contact her through e-mail at jane.booth@in-silence.net.

ISBN 142512004-0